Coagulation for
CLS & MLT

MARY MICHELLE SHODJA, PHD, MS, CLS (ASCP)

Order this book online at www.trafford.com
or email orders@trafford.com

Most Trafford titles are also available at major online book retailers.

Print information available on the last page.

ISBN: 978-1-4907-8788-6

Because of the dynamic nature of the Internet, any web addresses or links contained in this book may have changed
since publication and may no longer be valid. The views expressed in this work are solely those of the author and do
not necessarily reflect the views of the publisher, and the publisher hereby disclaims any responsibility for them.

Our mission is to efficiently provide the world's finest, most comprehensive book publishing
service, enabling every author to experience success. To find out how to publish your book,
your way, and have it available worldwide, visit us online at www.trafford.com

Any people depicted in stock imagery provided by Thinkstock are models,
and such images are being used for illustrative purposes only.
Certain stock imagery © Thinkstock.

Trafford rev. 03/15/2018

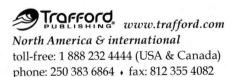

www.trafford.com
North America & international
toll-free: 1 888 232 4444 (USA & Canada)
phone: 250 383 6864 • fax: 812 355 4082

To my mother, for her sacrifices, this is for you.

To my cousin who is almost like a sister to me, Chona Aros, you are the most kind-hearted individual I know, thank you for your love and support. With deep gratitude to Christine Sy and my bestfriends, Anna Hamilton and Helena Pangan, thank you for your friendship of 25+ years.

"Success is not final, failure is not fatal: It is the courage to continue that counts"
Winston Churchill

To laboratory students and fellow laboratorians, never forget what you learned and never stop learning new things.
The Author

Preface

This manual is the fifth of a series of 20 manuals that the author was commissioned to write for the Medical Laboratory Technology (MLT) training program in Diamond Bar, California that was granted approval as a training facility in 2009 by the State Department of Health and Human Services. In writing these manuals, the author strived to adhere to the strict guidelines of the State of California's requirements for the MLT program.

The author revised these manuals to serve 3 purpose: as the primary textbooks for the 6-month MLT training program, as reviewers for Clinical Laboratory Scientists (CLSs) preparing for the CLS Licensure or Certification, and as a continuing education materials for CLSs and MLTs as a requirement for license renewal.

The author wrote these manuals in an outline form for easy reading and understanding and free from the constraint of a formal textbook. The author's intention is to speak to the reader from the actual clinical laboratory bench than from the classroom.

The Coagulation for CLS and MLT only discussed the most common coagulation disorders encountered in the clinical laboratory and is not intended as a replacement to the actual textbooks currently being employed in the CLS program.

Also by Mary Michelle Shodja, PhD, MS, CLS (ASCP)

Bacteriology for CLS & MLT
Hematology for CLS & MLT
Parasitology for CLS & MLT
Mycology for CLS & MLT
Virology for CLS & MLT
Urinalysis and Body Fluids for CLS & MLT
Routine Chemistry for CLS & MLT
Special Chemistry for CLS & MLT
Toxicology for CLS & MLT
Serology – Immunoassays for CLS & MLT
Serology – ELISA Assays for CLS & MLT
Serology & Syphilis for CLS & MLT
Immunology for CLS & MLT
Blood Bank for CLS & MLT
Phlebotomy for CLS & MLT
Specimen Processing for CLS & MLT
Laboratory Safety for CLS & MLT
Total Quality Management I – Quality Assurance
Total Quality Management II – Quality Control

Contents

SECTION I: Introduction to Coagulation & Hemostasis

The vascular system consists of three types of blood vessels:
1. Arteries – blood vessels that carry blood away from the heart narrowing down into arterioles and carrying oxygenated blood to all cells
2. Veins – capillaries that widens to the blood vessels that carry blood towards the heart carrying deoxygenated blood from the tissues back to the lungs
3. Capillaries – the smallest blood vessels and connects arterioles and venules

Hemostasis

The process of forming the barrier to blood loss and maintain the blood in the fluid state is referred to as Hemostasis. A traumatic injury such as a cut to the skin, severed vessels or any other injury that results to bleeding triggers platelets and dissolved proteins in an insoluble mass of structural barrier that occludes the injured tissue or vessel.

Primary Hemostasis
- Platelets interact with the injured vessels and with each other to form a plug called the Primary hemostatic plug that temporarily arrests the bleeding and is fragile. The plug forms in a specific sequence of steps:
  a. Platelet adhesion – first step in the primary hemostatic plug formation is the attachment of platelets to something besides other

platelets. Platelet adhesion to collagen will only occur with the help of Von Willebrand factor and glycoprotein 1b of the platelet membrane.

b. Activation – adhesion of platelets to collagen fibers triggers morphologic and functional changes known as activation. The activated platelets grow finger-like projections called pseudopodia which helps the platelet to move rapidly to the affected area and helps it to bind to collagen.

- ◦ Agonist – agent that induces platelet activation
  Thromboxane A2- synthesized from Prostaglandin H2 by Thromboxane-A Synthase produced by activated platelets, stimulates activation of new platelets as well as increases platelet aggregation
- ◦ Antagonist – agent that prevents platelet activation
  Aspirin – an antagonist, inhibits cyclooxygenase 1 and prevents formation of prostaglandin H2 and therefore Thromboxane A2

c. Aggregation – after platelet activation, platelet attaches to each other and aggregate.

- ◦ Primary aggregation – platelets adhere loosely to each other, if the stimulus of the agonist is weak, primary aggregation is reversible
- ◦ Secondary aggregation – takes a longer period of time and occurs as platelets start to release its own Adenosine diphosphate (ADP) and other granule contents and to synthesize Thromboxane A2

- Fibrinogen and extracellular calcium – needed for aggregation to occur
- Glycoprotein IIb/IIIa receptors – needed for platelet aggregation
  > Note: Glanzmann's Thrombocythemia – a disorder wherein there is a lack of Glycoprotein IIb/IIIa receptors

d. Secretion – following adhesion, activation and aggregation, platelets begin to discharge granule contents into the surrounding area and this process is known as secretion or release

LABORATORY TESTS FOR PRIMARY HEMOSTASIS
1. Platelet counts
   - Manual Method – 2 commonly described procedures are Rees and Ecker using Brilliant Cresyl Blue and Brecker-Cronkite using Ammonium Oxalate. Manual methods are performed by diluting a sample of whole blood, counting the platelets in an aliquot (using the Neubauer Hemocytometer) and calculating the number per liter.
   - Estimated platelet count – a peripheral blood smear is stained with Wright's stain and evaluated. The number of platelets (x 10^3) can be estimated by multiplying the average number seen on 100x oil immersion by 15 or 20 (depending on the microscope being used). Normal platelet count has between 8-10 platelets per field using 100x oil immersion.
   - Automated platelet count – part of the regular Complete Blood Count (CBC)

2. Platelet function evaluation
    a. Bleeding Time – in vivo measurement of primary hemostasis. 3 methods for performing this tests are:
        ◦ Duke Method
        ◦ Ivy Method
        ◦ Mielke Template Method

    The above methods differ in the site and manner of making the incision. Normal bleeding time is <15 minutes, abnormal is > 15 minutes. Bleeding Time should not be performed on patients who have ingested aspirin containing products in the past 7 days.

    b. Platelet Aggregation Test
        ◦ an invitro test of the ability of the platelets to aggregate with certain agonists. This test may be indicated in patients who have prolonged bleeding times in the presence of normal platelet counts.
        ◦ Aggregation is measured spectrophotometrically and recorded by a plaletet aggregometer. Aggregating reagents commonly used are ADP, epinephrine, collagen and ristocetin.
        ◦ Platelet aggregation is a useful aid in the diagnosis of Von Willebrand's Disease, Bernard-Soulier and Glanzmann's Thromobocythemia.
        ◦ Patients should be aspirin-free one week before the test

    c. Cold Retraction Test
        ◦ Retraction of the blood clot is explained as a result of spontaneous contraction of material liberated from the

thrombocytes during the first phase of viscous (in cold temperature) metamorphosis.

- ◦ Viscous metamorphosis of the blood platelets is defined to include all the changes observed in these cells during blood coagulation, the result of which is the liberation of various platelet factors.
- ◦ It was shown that the factors involved in the formation and action of thromboplastin includes antihemophilic globulin, factors V, VII, IX and calcium

Secondary Hemostasis
- Insoluble strands of fibrin get deposited on the primary plug to make it strong and stable. Generation of this fibrin strands involves a series of complex biochemical reactions
- Secondary hemostasis occurs when soluble plasma proteins, called coagulation factors interact in a series of complex enzymatic reactions to convert the soluble protein Fibrinogen to insoluble Fibrin through a cascade or waterfall-like series of reactions
- Both primary and secondary hemostasis is necessary for normal clot formation

PRIMARY AND SECONDARY HEMOSTASIS DEFICIENCIES:
- Primary Hemostasis deficiencies – usually produces small pinpoint hemorrhages beneath the skin called petechiae and bleeding from mucous membranes
- Secondary Hemostasis deficiencies – produce ecchymosis (large bruises) and more serious deep hemorrhages into joints and body cavities

- Natural inhibitors or regulators – limit the proteolytic (degrading/digesting) activity of the activated clotting factors

Once the injury is repaired, clots that were formed are no longer needed and needs to be dissolved.
Fibrinolysis
- The breakdown of the fibrin or clot

SECTION II: Automated Coagulation Analyzers

Most automated analyzers for specific clinical use in coagulation and/or fibrinolysis testing include both direct hemostatic measurements and calculated parameters. The principle behind most automated coagulation analyzers is spectrophotometric to detect clot formation.

Automated coagulation analyzers are capable of performing the following tests:
1. Protime (PT) & Fibrinogen
2. Activated Partial Thromboplastin Time (APTT)
3. Thrombin Time (TT)
4. Extrinsic Pathway Factors (II, V, VII, X)
5. Intrinsic Pathway Factors (VIII, IX, XI, XII)
6. Single factors (II, V, VII, VIII, IX, X, XI, XII)

Specimen requirement: Whole blood collected in sodium citrate with a 9:1 proportion of blood and anticoagulant.

PT, PTT and TT are reported in seconds
Fibrinogen levels are reported as either mg/dL or g/L
INR = International Normalized Ratio is automatically calculated by the analyzer by using the following formula:

$$\frac{\text{PT of patient}}{\text{PT of reference plasma}} = (\text{Ratio})^{\text{ISI}}$$

Protime Reagent
Tissue Thromboplastin (usually from a rabbit's plasma) is a lipoprotein found in many mammalian tissues. In the presence of calcium ions, thromboplastin is capable of activating the extrinsic pathway of coagulation (II, V, VII, X).

Fibrinogen Reagent
Thrombin acts on fibrinogen an acute-phase reactive protein and convert it to fibrin. The amount of converted fibrin is proportional to the amount of fibrinogen.

Activated Partial Thromboplastin Reagent + Calcium Chloride
Contains synthetic phospholipids, buffer and preservatives is capable of evaluating the extrinsic and common pathways of the coagulation cascade which includes factors I, II, V, VIII, IX, X, XI and XII.

Most automated analyzers uses the same patient to reagent proportion:

Protime
    100 ul of patient plasma (full blue top tube, Sodium Citrate)
    + 200 ul Thromboplastin reagent (Rabbit plasma)
    Perform test at 37⁰C

Fibrinogen
    100 ul of patient plasma (full blue top tube, Sodium Citrate)
    + 100 ul thrombin
    Perform test at 37⁰C

Note: Quantitation is obtained by comparing the clotting time in seconds/fibrinogen concentrations.

Activated Partial Thromboplastin Time
    100 ul pt. plasma (full blue top tube, Sodium Citrate) incubate 1-2 min at 37°C
    + 100 ul APTT Reagent (colloidal silica dispersion with synthetic phospholipids, buffer and preservatives) incubate 3 minutes at 37°C
    + 100 ul Calcium Chloride
    Perform test at 37°C

SECTION III: Coagulation Factors

- Majority of the coagulation factors are synthesized in the liver and a few are made by monocytes, endothelial cells and megakaryocytes. The coagulation process has traditionally been divided into three pathways (intrinsic, extrinsic and common) based on the mode and sequence of coagulation protein activation in vitro.
- The coagulation factors can be divided into three groups depending on their physical properties:
    a. Prothrombin Group or Vitamin K dependent factors – includes II, VII, IX and X. Vitamin K is found in some vegetables, oils and leafy plants. It is also synthesized in the gut by various bacteria. It is a fat soluble vitamin.
    b. Fibrinogen Group – includes I, V, VIII and XIII – this group of factors is also referred to as the consumable group because they are consumed during the formation of fibrin and therefore absent from serum during formation of clot
    c. Contact Group – includes XI and XII as well as plasma proteins, Prekallikrein, and High Molecular Weight Kininogens (HMWK)

Table 1: List of Coagulation Factors:

Coagulation Factor	Preferred Descriptive Name	Synonyms
I	Fibrinogen	
II	Prothrombin	
III	Tissue Factor	Thromboplastin
IV	Ionic Calciums	
V	Proaccelerin	Labile Factor
VII	Proconvertin	Stable Factor
VIII	Anti-hemophilic Factor (AHF)	Anti-hemophiliac factor
IX	Plasma Thromboplastin Component (PTC)	Christmas Factor
X	Stuart Factor	Power Factor
XI	Plasma Thromboplastin antecedent (PTA)	
XII	Hageman Factor	Glass Factor
XIII	Fibrin Stabilizing Factor	
	Prekallikrein	Fletcher Factor
	High Molecular Weight Kininogen	Fitzgerald Factor
	Platelet Factor 3	

SECTION IV: Coagulation Cascade

Figure 1: Coagulation Cascade

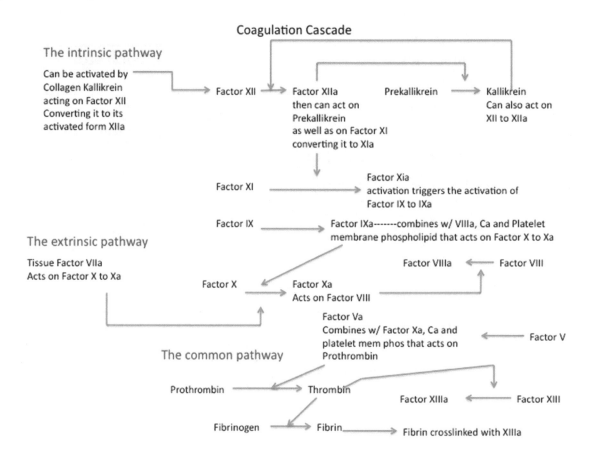

NOTE:
- When a factor becomes activated, a lower case "a" appears after the numeral

Physiological (In vivo) Coagulation Cascade – describes the very complex step-by-step process that occurs in the body when a blood vessel is injured. Several special proteins known as coagulation factors are activated one after the other in a "cascade" effect. The end result is a blood clot that creates a barrier over the injury site, protecting it until it heals. The process also involves a feedback system that regulates clot formation in the body so that clots are removed when the injury site is healed.

In vitro Coagulation Cascade – occurs when coagulation testing is performed in the laboratory. A sample of blood is tested by adding substances that begin the coagulation process and the time that it takes for the sample to begin to clot is measured.

INTRINSIC PATHWAY – components are all contained within the blood stream, hence the name "intrinsic"and includes factors VIII, IX, XI, XII, HMKW and Pre-kallikrein. The intrinsic factors in the order of the reaction are:
1. XII
2. Prekallikrein
3. HMWK
4. XI
5. IX
6. VIII
7. X
8. V
9. Prothrombin (II)
10. Fibrinogen (I)

XII -> XIIa activates Kallikrein (a subgroup of serine protease family and cleaves peptide bonds in proteins, liberates kinins from Kininogens), V to Va and factor XI->XIa

XIa->activate IX to IXa
Occurring simultaneously, Kallikrein is activating both Factor VIII to VIIIa and XIII to XIIIa

IXa, VIIIa, Calcium (IV) and Phospholipid activates X to Xa

Xa in turn also activates VIII to VIIIIa

EXTRINSIC PATHWAY (Tissue Factor Pathway) – extrinsic because the activation pathway requires a factor that does not circulate in the blood - involves factor I, II, V, VII, X, a CofactorTissue Factor (III). The extrinsic factors in the order of the reactions are:
1. VII + TF (III)
2. X
3. V
4. Prothrombin
5. Fibrinogen

Tissue Factor (III) acts as a cofactor with VIIa-> activates X to Xa

ENTERS THE COMMON PATHWAY

Common Pathway – includes three reactions each representing a key rate-limiting step in the cascade:

1. X – by products of intrinsic (VIIIa, IXa, Platelet Factor 3, Calcium) and extrinsic pathways (VIIa, Tissue Factor, Calcium)
2. Prothrombin (II) – conversion to Thrombin by activated factor X, activated Factor V, PF3 and Calcium
3. Fibrinogen (I) – cleaved to fibrin by Thrombin

Xa, Va, Calcium (IV) and Phospholipids (PL) converts Prothrombin to Thrombin

Thrombin converts Fibrinogen to Fibrin

XIIIa (previously activated by Kallikrein) stabilizes the fibrin clot

SECTION V: Laboratory Tests

THE MOST COMMON TESTS FOR COAGULATION SCREENING ARE PT AND APTT (PTT)

Prothrombin Time (PT) – measures the factors that are part of the extrinsic and common pathways (VII, X, V, II and Fibrinogen). In this test, an optimal concentration of tissue thromboplastin is added to the plasma providing the tissue factor necessary to activate the extrinsic pathway.

Partial Thromboplastin Time (PTT) or Activated Partial Thromboplastin Time (APTT) – measures those protein factors that are part of the cascade often referred to as intrinsic and common pathways (XII, XI, IX, VIII, X, V, II and Fibrinogen) as well as Prekallikrein (PK) and High Molecular Weight Kininogen (HMWK). This test measures all factors except VII and XIII. In this test, an activator substance such as Kaloin, celite or ellagic acid is incubated with plasma to activate the contact factors followed by the addition of a phospholipid substitute for platelets and calcium.

Thrombin Time (TT) – measures only the conversion of fibrinogen to fibrin. In this test thrombin is added to citrated plasma and the time for a clot to form is measured.

Russell's Viper Venom – obtained from the East Indian Viper contains a protease similar to factor VIIa that can selectively and directly activate factor X. This test was used primarily to differentiate factor VII deficiency from Factor X deficiency

Fibrin Degradation Products (FDPs) – assays are available based on the reaction of monoclonal antibodies with specific fibrin derivatives.

- ◦ If antiserum to fibrinogen fragments D and E is used, a positive result may be obtained with fibrinogen degradation products as well as FDPs
- ◦ If antiserum is highly specific to an antigen on D-Dimers, the test will be positive only if fibrin degradation has occurred, thus the D-Dimer test is a specific marker for plasmin degradation of fibrin

FACTOR DEFICIENCY STUDIES

In able to find out what factor is missing on an individual that is having coagulation disorder, it is important to perform factor studies. The following could be used to perform factor deficiency studies:

- Normal Plasma – should have all factors present
- Aged Normal Plasma (old plasma) – factors present includes I,II,VII,IX, X, XI, XII and absent (V and VIII)
- Normal Serum – factors present includes VII, IX, X, XI, XII and absent I, II, V, VIII and XIII
- BaSO$_4$ or Al(OH)$_2$ adsorbed plasma – have the following factors present I,V,VIII,XI,XI,XIII and absent I, VII, IX, X

SPECIALIZED COAGULATION TESTS (activators and inhibitors)

Coagulation is controlled by:
- a. Blood flow
- b. Liver clearance of activated factors

c. Feedback inhibition
d. Biochemical inhibitors (naturally occurring anticoagulants) – soluble plasma proteins that regulate the enzymatic reactions of serine proteases preventing the initiation or amplification of the clotting cascade. These protease inhibitors include:
   ◦ Anti-thrombin III – single chain glycoprotein produced in the liver, endothelial cells and possibly the megakaryocytes and by far the most important inhibitor of coagulation inhibiting thrombin.
   ◦ Heparin cofactors – inhibits IIa and a cofactor for heparin and dermatan sulfate
   ◦ Tissue Pathway Inhibitor (TFPI) – can reversibly inhibit Xa and Thrombin
   ◦ Protein C and S
     Protein C – a vitamin K dependent anticoagulant that degrades Va and VIIIa. The optimal activation of protein C requires a cofactor and calcium. The inhibitor activity of activated protein C is enhanced by another vitamin K dependent protein, protein S
     Protein S – acts as a cofactor of Protein C
   ◦ C1 inactivator – inhibits XIa, XIIa and plasma kallikrein
e. Fibrinolytic dissolution of fibrin
   ◦ Plasminogen – is a circulating zymogen that is converted to the active enzyme plasmin. Activators of Plasminogen can be found in blood (intrinsic) and in most tissues (extrinsic). In addition, some substances not normally present in the blood during the coagulation and fibrinolytic process can gain access to the circulation in pathologic states and can activate plasminogen

- ◦ Activators can be extrinsic (urokinase, tissue plasminogen activator, streptokinase) or intrinsic (kallikrein)
- ◦ Plasmin – an important enzyme present in the blood that degrades many blood plasma proteins notably fibrin clots→Fibrin Degradation products (FDPs) which are cleared by the liver
- ◦ Fibrin fragments (FDPs) – if elevated can exert anticoagulant effect on the clotting system and can also interfere with primary hemostasis by inhibiting platelet aggregation

The clotting of blood and subsequent dissolution of the clot through fibrinolysis is an intricately regulated process that is kept in balance by the interaction of activators and inhibitors. If this balance is upset by a deficiency of or an inappropriate activation of activators or inhibitors, thrombosis or bleeding may occur.

SECTION VI: Coagulation Disorders

Abnormalities in the PT are seen in the condition other than congenital factor deficiencies. The PT are prolonged in:

a. Liver disease and obstructive jaundice
b. Oral anticoagulants depress the Vitamin K-dependent synthesis of the Prothrombin Group (II, VII, IX, X). Note: Factor VII have the shortest half-life of these four factors
c. PT is the test of choice in monitoring Coumadin treatment of thrombotic conditions

Abnormal APTT (PTT) suggests abnormality in the intrinsic or common pathways and like PT is not sensitive to mild factor deficiencies. When PT and PTT are abnormal, the possibility of heparin contamination should be considered and could be eliminated by performing a thrombin time and a reptilase time. Heparin will prolong the thrombin time but the reptilase time is unaffected. Heparin contamination can also be ruled out by performing a heparin neutralization step with protamine sulfate and repeating the PTT test; if the test becomes normal then there was heparin contamination and the specimen should be recollected.

Fibrinogen deficiency, dysfibrinogenemia or the presence of circulating inhibitors such as heparin, plasmin and FDPs – indicated by the prolonged TT. TT can be used to monitor heparin therapy or detect heparin contamination since heparin acts as an anticoagulant by inhibiting thrombin.

Decrease Levels of Anti-thrombin III (ATIII) may be hereditary or acquired and are associated with venous thrombosis. Hereditary ATIII deficiency is found in 2-3% of individuals with venous thromboembolisms. Acquired deficiency of ATIII have been associated with oral contraceptives, surgery, septicemia, and liver disease.

Protein C or S deficiency – associated with venous thrombosis and are at risk for development of thromboembolisms

INHERITED DISORDERS

Von Willebrand Disease (vWD) – arises from a qualitative or quantitative deficiency of Von Willebrand Factor (VWF), a multimeric protein that is required for protein adhesion. The various types of vWD present with varying degrees of bleeding tendency, usually in the form of easy bruising, nose bleeds and bleeding gums. Women may experience heavy menstrual periods and blood loss during childbirth. Four types had been described (Type 1, 2, 3 and platelet type).

- VWF and Factor VIII are two functionally and antigenically separate proteins. VWF serves as the Factor VIII carrier protein molecule but the primary function is to participate in platelet adhesion to subendothelial collagen in regions of high blood flow rate and high shear force, as in arteries and arterioles.
- Treatment: vWD usually has mild symptoms and treatment of localized hemorrhages is accomplished by the use of pressure and ice packs. In multiple hemorrhage situations, various combinations of estrogen and Desmopressin Acetate (DDAVP).

- Patients with Hemophilia "A" have decreased plasma factor VIII activity but their VWF is normal so they have normal platelet function and normal VWF by immunologic tests
- VWF Disease – have template bleeding time that measures the platelet function as abnormal not because the platelets are abnormal but because in the absence of VWF, the platelets cannot adhere to collagen and initiate the series of reaction that lead to formation of primary homeostatic plug. VWF Disease is the most common inherited bleeding disorder in humans.
    - Platelet aggregation test results will be normal for ADP, collagen and epinephrine but abnormal or fails to aggregate with ristocetin
    - PT, Platelet count and TT are normal
    - PTT is prolonged

Hemophilias – congenital single-coagulation-factor deficiencies marked by anatomic bleeding. Hemophilias occur in 1 in 10,000 individuals, of these 85% are factor VIII deficient, 14% are factor IX deficient and 1% are factor XI deficient.

Factor Deficiencies
1. Factor VIII deficiency or Classic Hemophilia or Hemophilia A– the International Committee on Thrombosis and Hemostasis defines Factor VIII as the protein that circulates in the plasma and functions in the intrinsic pathway of fibrin formation. Synthesized in the liver.
    - Hemophilia A inheritance is sex-linked, males experience bleeding symptoms but not female carriers
    - Hemophilia A causes anatomic bleeds with deep muscle and joint hemorrhages, hematomas, easy bruising, wound oozing following trauma or surgery and bleeding into the central

nervous system, peritoneum, retroperitoneal, gastrointestinal tract and kidneys

- The properties of Factor VIII are:

a. VIII:C – is the activity of factor in fibrin formation, also called the procoagulant or coagulation activity.

b. VIIIAg – antigenic quality of Factor VIII

   - In the absence of family history, abnormal bleeding in the neonatal period, such as intracranial bleeding at birth, bleeding from the umbilical stump, postcircumcision bleeding, hematuria, or easy bruising is a sign
   - The severity of Hemophilia A is inversely proportional to the Factor VIII activity, activity level of 0-2 U/dL is severe, levels of 2-6 U/dL is moderate and 6-30 U/dL is mild
   - Diagnosis begins with laboratory testing following the birth of an infant to a mother who has a family history of hemophilia. PT, PTT, TT and single factor assays
   - PT and TT are normal
   - PTT is prolonged
   - Factor VIII activity is <50 U/dL
   - Treatment: Therapeutic Factor VIII twice a day intramuscular or intranasal administration of Desmopressin Acetate (trade name DDAVP) or intravenous factor VIII concentrate for severe hemophiliacs

Hemophilia A Factor VIII inhibitor

- Alloantibody inhibitors of factor VIII arise in response to treatment in approximately 20% of severe hemophiliacs and 3% of moderate hemophiliacs

- Factor VIII inhibitors are generally immunoglobulin G4 isotype, non-complement fixing warm-reacting antibodies
- Factor VIII inhibitor is suspected when factor VIII activity fails to rise to the anticipated levels following concentrate administration
- Laboratory: Mixing studies detects inhibitors
- Patient's sample with a prolonged PTT is mixed with normal plasma that has a factor VIII level activity near 100% and incubated at 37^0C for 2 hours
- Absence of inhibitor= normal or almost normal level PTT
- Inhibitor present = Factor VIII in normal plasma gets neutralized and the PTT is prolonged

  Presence of Lupus anticoagulants (not warm reacting) may prolonged the PTT results
- Treatment: Load as much Factor VIII to neutralize the inhibitor or use Porcine factor VIII

2. Factor IX Deficiency – Hemophilia B- Christmas Disease – incidence in India equals that of Hemophilia A
   - Caused by deficiency in factor IX which is one of the vitamin K dependent
   - Sex-linked and ranges from mild to severe
   - Factor IX is the substrate for both factors XI and VII
   - Factor IX deficiency slows the coagulation process and causes anatomic bleeding similar to Hemophilia A
   - Laboratory: PT, PTT, TT and factor assays
   - PT and TT = normal

- ◦ PTT =prolonged
- ◦ Treatment: monoclonally purified factor IX concentrate

3. Factor XI Deficiency – Rosenthal Syndrome
   - ◦ Autosomal codominant with mild to moderate anatomic symptoms
   - ◦ Over 50% of the cases have been described in Ashkenazi Jews
   - ◦ Treatment: frequent infusion of Fresh Frozen Plasma during time of hemostatic challenges

4. Fibrinogen (Factor I) Deficiencies – 2 forms are inherited as autosomal recessive traits but both have PT, PTT and TT and bleeding time are prolonged
   - ◦ Afibrinogenemia – no fibrinogen
   - ◦ Hypofibrinogenemia – low fibrinogen
   - ◦ Treatment: Fibrinogen in the form of cryoprecipitate or Fresh Frozen Plasma (FFP)

5. Prothrombin (Factor II) Deficiency- extremely rare disease
   - ◦ PT, PTT are prolonged

6. Factor V Deficiency – Parahemophilia – extremely rare
   - ◦ PT, PTT are prolonged

7. Factor VII Deficiency
   - ◦ PTT, TT, platelet count and functions are normal
   - ◦ PT prolonged
   - ◦ Treatment: FFP or Prothrombin concentrates

8. Factor X Deficiency
    ◦ PT, PTT and Rusell's Viper Venom are prolonged
    ◦ Treatment: FFP

9. Factor XIII Deficiency
    ◦ Unable to form a stable clot
    ◦ Laboratory: Dissolution of clot with 5M urea – screening test
    ◦ A positive test with 5M urea is indicative of Factor XIII concentration of 0.005 U/ml or less

ACQUIRED DISORDERS

Disseminated Intravascular Coagulation (DIC)
    ◦ Condition in which the normal balance of hemostasis is altered allowing the uncontrolled inappropriate formation of fibrin within the blood vessels
    ◦ As fibrin is formed, several clotting proteins, especially fibrinogen are consumed at a faster rate than they are synthesized
    ◦ Platelets become caught within the fibrin mass
    ◦ As a result of the coagulation factor and platelet consumption and the presence of FDP, bleeding may occur at the same time
    ◦ Conditions most often associated with the development of DIC are:
    ◦ Infections
    ◦ Complications of pregnancy
    ◦ Neoplasms
    ◦ Snake bite
    ◦ Laboratory: Decrease in platelet count and decrease fibrinogen level as well as presence of FDP and Fibrin Split Products (FSP)

Vitamin K deficiency
- ◦ o   Needed by hepatic cells to complete the posttranslational alteration of factors II, VII, IX and X, protein C and S
- ◦ Sources of vitamin K are:
    Green, leafy vegetables in the diet
    Synthesis of bacteria in the gastrointestinal tract

Acquired Pathologic Inhibitors
Lupus-like anticoagulant (LLAC) – so called because it was discovered in patients with Systemic Lupus Erythematosus (SLE). Antibodies bind to phospholipids and proteins associated with the cell membrane and can interfere with blood clotting as well as in vitro tests of clotting factors. Lupus anticoagulants are also risk factors for thrombosis. Laboratory tests the presence of the antibody and usually employs ELISA.

ANTICOAGULANT THERAPY
1. Oral Coagulants
    a. Dicumarols
    b. Coumarins (Coumadin) – most commonly used, prevent thrombin generation by inhibiting vitamin K
    c. Indanediones
2. Heparin – acts on anti-thrombin III and inactivates the serine proteases. Heparin is used to treat thromboembolic disorders and pulmonary embolisms. Heparin is given intramuscularly or intravenously or subcutaneously

SECTION VII: Normal Values

Normal Coagulation values vary between laboratories. Below are commonly used normal values:

vWF – 0.5-1.0 mg/dL
Factor VIII activity >50 U/dL
PT: 11-15 seconds
INR: 0.8-1.2 ***calculated as [(INR= patient PT/Normal PT)[ISI]****
PTT: 30-45 seconds
TT: 10-15 seconds
Fibrinogen: 170-420 mg/dL

SECTION VIII: Critical Ranges

Critical values vary between laboratories. Below are commonly used critical ranges:

PT > 25 seconds
PTT > 65 seconds
Fibrinogen > 650 mg/dL

COAGULATION -WRITTEN EXAMINATION
(70 POINTS)

Student Name_____   Date_____

(Please circle the correct answer)

1. Platelet aggregation is a useful test for the diagnosis of the following diseases except:
   a. Von Willebrand Disease
   b. Factor VIII Disease
   c. Bernard-Soulier Disease
   d. Glanzmann's Disease

2. Please calculate the INR using the following data: Normal PT = 11.9 seconds, Patient PT = 15.1 seconds, ISI = 1.859

   INR = _____

3. The intrinsic pathway started with the activation of:
   a. IX
   b. X
   c. XI
   d. XII

4. A step in the formation of the primary hemostatic plug wherein platelets form finger-like projections called pseudopodia
   a. Adhesion
   b. Secretion
   c. Aggregation

     d. Activation

5. The following coagulation factors belong to the Fibrinogen Group except:
    a. I
    b. V
    c. VII
    d. VIII
    e. XIII

6. The PT test measures:
    a. VII, IX, X, II and Fibrinogen
    b. V, VII, X, II and Fibrinogen
    c. VII, X, V, II and Fibrinogen
    d. VII, XI, V, II and Fibrinogen

7. The patient had a normal PT and a prolonged PTT. One part patient plasma was added to one part normal plasma corrected the PTT. One part of patient plasma and one part of aged plasma prolonged the PTT. Knowing that the PT is normal what is the most likely factor that is deficient:
    a. II
    b. V
    c. VIII
    d. X

8. Normal bleeding time is:
    a. <20
    b. <15
    c. <10
    d. <5

9. We do not spontaneously coagulate because of the natural anti-coagulants that we produce. The following are all natural anti-coagulants except:
    a. Protein C and S
    b. Tissue Pathway Inhibitors
    c. C4 Inactivators
    d. Heparin cofactors
    e. Anti-thrombin III

10. A patient has a normal PT and prolonged PTT. Addition of normal plasma corrected the PTT. Addition of Aged plasma corrected the PTT. $BaSO_4$ did not correct the PTT. Which coagulation factor is the most likely to be deficient?
    a. VIII
    b. IX
    c. X
    d. XI

11. This is the first step in the formation of the primary hemostatic plug
    a. Adhesion
    b. Secretion
    c. Aggregation
    d. Activation

12. The following are plasminogen activators except:
    a. Streptokinase
    b. Plasmin
    c. Urokinase
    d. kallikrein

13. Heparin will prolong:
    a. PT

b. PTT

c. TT

d. Fibrinogen

14. A normal platelet count and a prolonged bleeding time is an indication that there is a problem in:

    a. Platelet activation

    b. Platelets adhesion

    c. Platelet secretion

    d. Platelet aggregation

15. The patient had a prolonged PT and PTT results. Addition of Normal Plasma corrected both. Addition of Aged plasma did not correct both. Addition of $BaSO_4$ corrected both. What is the most likely coagulation factor that is deficient?

    a. V

    b. VII

    c. VIII

    d. IX

16. The following acts as agonists:

    a. Thromboxane A2

    b. Prostaglandin H2

    c. Aspirin

    d. Cyclooxygenase

    e. a and b

    f. a and c

    g. a and d

    h. b and c

    i. b and d

j. c and d

17. A normal PT, and TT and prolonged PTT and bleeding time and a normal Factor VIII activity may indicate Von Willebrand Disease
    a. True
    b. False

18. Assays that contain anti-serum to fibrinogen fragments D and E will react with both fibrinogen degradation products and fibrin degradation products
    a. True
    b. False

19. The following coagulation factors belong to the Contact Group except:
    a. IX
    b. XI
    c. XII
    d. Prekallikrein
    e. High Molecular Weight Kininogen

20. Changes to the blood platelets after exposure to cold is the basis of the cold retraction test:
    a. True
    b. False

21. The blood vessel that carry blood away from the heart
    a. Arteries
    b. Capillaries
    c. Lymphatics
    d. Veins

22. A step in the formation of the primary hemostatic plug wherein platelets attaches to each other

a. Adhesion

b. Aggregation

c. Secretion

d. Activation

23. A normal platelet count usually has _____ platelets/100x oil immersion

    a. 5-8

    b. 8-10

    c. 15-20

    d. 20-30

24. The PTT test measures the following:

    a. XII, XI, IX, VIII, X, V, II and Fibrinogen

    b. XII, X, IX, VII, V, II and Fibrinogen

    c. XIII, IX, VIII, V, II and Fibrinogen

    d. XII, XI, IX, VII, X, V, II and Fibrinogen

25. Hemophilia A will have Factor VIII activity

    a. <20

    b. <30

    c. <40

    d. <50

26. Defects attributed to primary hemostasis usually produce small, pinpoint hemorrhages while those attributed to secondary hemostatis produce large and deeper bruises

    a. True

    b. False

27. The following coagulation factors are found in the extrinsic pathway except:

    a. III

b. VII

c. X

d. XII

28. Presence of FDP and FSP is diagnostic for Disseminated Intravascular Coagulation:

    a. True

    b. False

29. Please match (1 point each)

_____ Factor I	a.	Proaccelerin
_____ Factor II	b.	Tissue Factor
_____ Factor III	c.	Anti-Hemophilic Factor
_____ Factor IV	d.	Stuart Factor
_____ Factor V	e.	Fibrinogen
_____ Factor VII	f.	Plasma Thromboplastin Antecedent
_____ Factor VIII	g.	Hageman Factor
_____ Factor IX	h.	Ionic Calcium
_____ Factor X	i.	Fibrin Stabilizing Factor
_____ Factor XI	j.	Christmas Factor
_____ Factor XII	k.	Prothrombin
_____ Factor XIII	l.	Proconvertin

30. Primary hemostasis is the formation of the stabilized clot while secondary hemostasis is the formation of the unstable clot

    a. True

    b. False

31. The smallest blood vessel and serves as a connector for 2 major vessels:

    a. Arteries

    b. Capillaries

c. Lymphatics

d. Veins

32. The following coagulation factors are vitamin K dependent except:

    a. I

    b. II

    c. VII

    d. IX

    e. X

33. To differentiate a true Hemophilia A from Factor VIII inhibitor, a mixing study is performed with normal plasma. Presence of Factor VIII inhibitor will have what result with PTT mixing with normal plasma?

    a. Normal

    b. Prolonged

34. Hemophilia B or Christmas Disease is Vitamin K dependent

    a. True

    b. False

35. The following components are required for platelet aggregation:

    a. Calcium

    b. Fibrinogen

    c. Glycoprotein Ib/IIa

    d. Glycoprotein IIb/IIIa

    e. a, b and c

    f. a, b and d

    g. a, c and d

    h. b, c and d

36. Classic Hemophilia is:

    a. Hemophilia A

b. Hemophilia B

c. Christmas Factor

d. Hemophilia C

37. The enzyme responsible for the dissolution of the fibrin once the injury is repaired is:

    a. Urokinase

    b. Streprokinase

    c. Plasmin

    d. kallikrein

38. The following coagulation factors are found in the common pathway except:

    a. I

    b. II

    c. X

    d. XI

39. The reagent for Protime is:

    a. Colloidal silica

    b. Thromboplastin

    c. Plasminogen

    d. Thrombin

40. The Russell's Viper Venom Test can directly activate Factor X and differentiates it from factor _____ deficiency:

    a. V

    b. VI

    c. VII

    d. VIII

41. If the patient's PT is prolonged and PTT is normal and addition of $BaSO_4$ did not correct the PT, what is the most likely coagulation factor that is deficient?
    a. I
    b. II
    c. V
    d. VII
    e. X
42. What would be the expected result of the Russell's Viper Venom Test (RVVT)?
    a. Normal
    b. Prolonged
43. Calcium is added on which assay:
    a. PT
    b. PTT
    c. TT
    d. Fibrinogen
44. D-Dimer test is the test of choice for the presence of Fibrin Degradation Products because it does not react with Fibrinogen Degradation Products
    a. True
    b. False
45. The vitamin K dependent anticoagulant that degrades Va and VIIIa is:
    a. Anti-thrombin III
    b. Tissue Pathway inhibitor
    c. Heparin cofactors
    d. Protein C

46. A step in the formation of primary hemostatic plug whereby granule contents are release in the surrounding area:
    a. Adhesion
    b. Aggregation
    c. Secretion
    d. activation
47. Thrombin Time measures the conversion of thrombin to fibrin
    a. True
    b. False
48. The extrinsic pathway starts with the activation of factor VII with:
    a. Tissue Cofactor
    b. Factor IX
    c. Calcium
    d. Plasminogen
49. The following coagulation factors are found in the intrinsic pathway except:
    a. V
    b. VIII
    c. IX
    d. XI
    e. XII
50. The blood vessel that carries blood towards the heart
    a. Arteries
    b. Capillaries
    c. Veins
    d. Lymphatics

51. Heparin contamination could be eliminated by performing a thromobin time and a reptilase test. Heparin contamination will have the following results:
   a. Thrombin normal, reptilase prolonged
   b. Thrombin prolonged, reptilase normal
   c. Thrombin and reptilase normal
   d. Thrombin and reptilase prolonged

52. Von Willebrand Disease will have normal platelet aggregation on the following except:
   a. Collagen
   b. Epinephrine
   c. Ristocetin
   d. ADP

53. Lupus anticoagulant will prolonged PT
   a. True
   b. False

54. Over 50% of the Factor XI Deficiency is seen among:
   a. Orthodox Jews
   b. Ashkenazi Jews
   c. East Indians
   d. Sephardic Jews

55. Factor I deficiency is treated with:
   a. Thawed Plasma
   b. Platelets
   c. Fresh Frozen Plasma
   d. Cryoplatelets

56. Factor X deficiency will have the following tests prolonged except:

a. PT

b. PTT

c. TT

d. RVVT

57. The 5M urea is a screening test for:

a. Factor II

b. Factor X

c. Factor XII

d. Factor XIII

58. A disease called Parahemophilia is associated to what deficient factor?

a. II

b. V

c. VII

d. X

59. Factor II deficiency is extremely rare and will have a:

a. Prolonged PT and normal PTT

b. Normal PT and prolonged PTT

c. Prolonged PT and PTT

d. Normal PT and PTT

Answer key Coagulation Written Examination
70 points

1. B	21. A	40. C
2. 1.6	22. B	41. D
3. D	23. B	42. B
4. D	24. A	43. B
5. C	25. D	44. A
6. C	26. A	45. D
7. C	27. D	46. D
8. B	28. A	47. B
9. C	29. E, K, B, H, A, L, C, J,	48. A
10. B	D,F, G, I	49. A
11. A	30. B	50. C
12. B	31. B	51. B
13. B	32. A	52. C
14. D	33. B	53. B
15. A	34. A	54. B
16. F	35. F	55. C
17. A	36. A	56. C
18. A	37. C	57. D
19. A	38. D	58. B
20. A	39. B	59. C

Afterword

In a perfect world, after their clinical rotation, CLSs and MLTs will be working in all four areas of study of medical technology or clinical science (Microbiology, Chemistry, Hematology and Immunohematology), retain all that they know and live and work happily ever after. But as we all know that is far from the case, more frequently than not, a CLS or MLT will be stuck in one or two specialized area of study. Coagulation is a unique sub-specialty of the department of Hematology and in most hospitals is limited to the testing of PT, PTT and fibrinogen. The specialized tests in coagulation is done exclusively in the large reference laboratories because these tests are not frequently ordered and maintaining reagents for testing is not cost effective for most hospitals. CLSs who had been away from the hematology and coagulation department for a period of time or never had the chance to work in a specialized coagulation department will need a good refresher course before venturing into these departments. This manual does not claim that it will boost someone's confidence overnight or claim to have all the answers, but instead this manual serves as a guide to re-discovering what one previously knew.

This manual is also directed towards CLS and MLT students at or nearing their clinical rotation as well as those taking the CLS and MLT State or National licenses.

My hope is that this manual will serve its purpose and be a source of confidence to those who are contemplating to work in the hematology or specialized coagulation department as a newbee or someone who had been away from it for a period of time.

Glossary

ACUTE PHASE REACTIVE PROTEINS – proteins that are present in elevated or decreased levels during trauma, inflammation or disease

AGGREGATION – a phenomenon wherein cells intermixed causing it to "aggregate"

ANTICOAGULANT – agents that prevent clotting

BRILIANT CRESYL BLUE – a supravital stain (stains live cells) classified as an oxazine dye

COLLAGEN – any group of fibrous proteins that occur in vertebrates as the chief constituent of connective tissue fibrils and in bones and yield gelatin and glue upon boiling with water

COUMADIN – used for preparation of warfarin, a blood thinner

CYCLOOXYGENASE 1 – or prostaglandin-endoperoxide synthase, is an enzyme that is responsible for formation of prostanoids such as thromboxane and prostaglandin

DERMATAN SULFATE – a naturally occurring glycosaminoglycan found mostly in the skin and connective tissue

DICUMAROL – an anticoagulant that acts in the liver to block synthesis of vitamin K and vitamin K dependent factors

DUKE METHOD – a method of testing for bleeding time wherein the patient is pricked with a special needle or lancet on the fingertip continually wiping the blood with the filter paper every 15 seconds and ending when bleeding ceases

EPINEPHRINE - a sympathomimetric hormone that is the principal blood-pressure raising hormone secreted by the medulla of the adrenal glands.

GLYCOPROTEIN – a conjugated protein in which the nonprotein group is a carbohydrate

HEPARIN – a mucopolysaccharide sulfuric ester that is found especially in the liver and lungs that prolongs the clotting time of blood

INDANEDIONE – any of a group of synthetic anticoagulant derived from 1,3-indanedione

IN VITRO – outside of the living body and in artificial environment

IVY METHOD – a method of testing for bleeding time wherein a blood pressure cuff is placed on the upper arm and inflated to 40mmHg. A lancet is used to make a shallow incision that is 1 mm deep on the underside of the forearm. A filter paper is used to wipe the blood and ending when bleeding ceases.

LUPUS ANTICOAGULANT – an antiphospholipid antibody found in association with Systemic Lupus Erythematosus (SLE)

MEGAKARYOCYTES – a large cell that has a lobulated nucleus, is found especially in the bone marrow and is the source of blood platelets

METAMORPHOSIS – a change of physical form, structure or substance

MIELKE TEMPLATE METHOD – a method of testing for bleeding time that is a modification of the Ivy method, the difference is mainly the employment of a blade that instead of a prick or a lancet

NEUBAUER HEMOCYTOMETER – is a thick cell counter crystal slide the size of a glass slide (30 x 70 mm but 4mm thick) with a 3 x 3 counting grid. The grid has 9 square subdivisions of 1mm width.

PERITONEUM – the smooth transparent serous membrane that lines the cavity of the abdomen of a mammal and is folded inward over the abdominal and pelvic viscera

PLASMA – the fluid part of blood that consists of water and its dissolved constituents

PLATELETS – non-nucleated disk-shaped cells formed in the megakaryocyte and found in the blood of all mammals

PROSTAGLAND H2 – a cyclic endoperoxide intermediate produced by the action of cyclooxigenase on arachidonic acid

PSEUDOPODIA – a dynamic actin-rich extension of the surface of an animal cell used for locomotion or prehension of food

REPTILASE TIME - clotting time of plasma mixed with a thrombin solution. It is a measure of the conversion of fibrinogen to fibrin

RETROPEROTENEAL – situated behind the peritoneum

RISTOCETIN – an antibiotic mixture of two components, A and B contained from Nocardia lurida causing platelet aggregarion and blood coagulation

THROMBOCYTES – another name for platelets

THROMBOXANE A2 – an unstable intermediate between prostaglandin endoperoxides and thromboxane B2, a potent inducer of platelet aggregation and causes vasoconstriction

THROMBOXANE A2 SYNTHASE – an enzyme found predominantly in platelet microsomes, catalyzes the conversion of prostaglandin endoperretoxides to thromboxane A2.

ZYMOGEN – an inactive precursor that is converted into an active enzyme by the action of an acid or another enzyme or by other means

References

Harmening, D. (2008). Clinical Hematology and Fundamentals of Hemostasis. 5th Edition. Philadelphia, PA. F.A. Davis Company.

Lee, G.R., Bithell, T.C., Foerster, J., Athens, J.W. and Lukens, J.N. (1993). Wintrobe's Clinical Hematology. 9th Edition. Philadelphia, PA. Lea & Febiger.

https://www.merriam-webster.com/

www.online-medical-dictionary.org/

About the Author

Mary Michelle Shodja earned her Bachelors of Science Degree in Medical Technology in 1992 from California State University (CSU) Dominguez Hills in Carson, California. She took her medical technology clinical year training from the Southern California Kaiser Permanente Medical Hospital and Regional Laboratory. She earned her Masters of Science Degree in Bioanalysis in 1995 from her alma mater CSU Dominguez Hills and her PhD in Epidemiology from Loma Linda University School of Public Health in 2017.

She gained Certifications in both the MLS American Society of Clinical Pathologists (ASCP) and CLS National Credentialing Agency (NCA) in 1993. Her professional career includes working in the Microbiology department at the Southern California Kaiser Permanente Regional Laboratory and as a generalist in various hospitals working in Hematology, Chemistry, Serology, Immunology and Blood Bank. She also worked for 4 years as a Microbiology laboratory instructor at Loma Linda University School of Allied Health.

Over the years she took on managerial, supervisory, teaching and other administrative and consultative work but her real passion lies in the clinical bench work and teaching. Earning her PhD in Epidemiology she plans to integrate her clinical laboratory knowledge to helping lower disease burdens globally.

Printed in the United States
By Bookmasters